ebb and flow

katie cecilia

other books by katie cecilia

growing

to the ones reaching the shore,

to the ones navigating the waves.

these tides move in cycles;

hope is not lost;

you are finding your way.

chapters

drift

i am good at writing about being sad.
probably because for a really long time
sadness was the only thing
that stayed with me.
sadness got me through
some of the hardest times in my life
and showed me
just how deep my heart can feel.
even after all this time,
despite how happy i may feel,
sadness is always the feeling
i write about first.

being sad is addictive; the cycle of better to worse keeps you stuck. sadness is predictable; it latches onto you like a leech, distorting every experience and draining your soul. you're tired, but warmth is unfamiliar. you adapt to the weight even when there are overlapping splinters and burns. you stay in what you know – even when it destroys you inside out.

i tell my mother that i want to be just like her,

she sighs and lists the things she hasn't achieved, as if
that would deter my mind.

i want her determination, how she moves mountains
when she puts her mind to it.

i want her strength, how she wades through seas
to reach the shore regardless of what waves are in her
way.

i want her care, how she pours into what she loves
and her ability to show up for the highs, lows and in-
betweens.

i want to be just like her,

a force of nature through every season.

comparison will have you thinking that your oceans of exploration are merely puddles in the street.

comparison will lead you to believe that someone else's shop window is more impressive than your field of sprouting seeds.

comparison will rob you of the joy in your progress as the distortion takes over how you look at the stepping stones of your life.

no matter how high you climb or soar, comparison will point out the height of the neighbouring mountains.

comparison will have you glancing over with a sigh in envy of the views they give, completely disregarding the blooming habitats that took you decades to create.

thank you for teaching me
that not all arms that wrap around me
intend to hurt,
that an embrace can
be for comfort
and an act
of utter care.

we were a candle burning at both ends. neither of us was happy, but neither of us had the courage to admit it then.

i brushed off your compliments and pulled away when we grazed hands. i knew i shouldn't have called you so late, but you were the only one to understand.

i saw you as my best friend;
you longed for something more.
i should have noticed the lingering.
i should have walked out the door.

we spent years scared of the change that would come once we finally acknowledged the truth.

it was time to address the elephant in the room.

i would never love you the way you wanted me to.

the evenings feel like
a teary-eyed deep sigh.
this is either where i blame the feeling on sleep
or finally admit
that i haven't felt myself
in a really,
   really
long
  time.

i have tried to fit
shoes a little too tight.

i have stayed with people
hoping i'd change my mind.

i have talked myself into
things i never wanted to do.

i have pushed for things
that fell right through.

no matter how much i tried
i couldn't deny my shape.

i was never meant for those boxes.

i was never built that way.

i openly tell people that i don't want children.

i use excuses like how they are expensive and how i have never felt a motherly instinct or how their fluctuating behaviour would get the best of me.

they usually nod and move on in conversation – brushing the comments off because they assume i will change my mind at twenty-eight.

i never say this when asked, but not being able to rewrite history by being better would be a devastation that would eat away at me.

i do not want children

because i am scared of not letting them be one.

it is our ritual that we send pictures of the weather to each other. this morning there are orange and pink hues here, the sun peeking behind the clouds. you say there's blue skies with potential rain where you are. it is in these moments that the distance doesn't seem as far. even with the miles and hour differences, we are still here, experiencing it all under the same sky.

ebb and flow

i am tearing my heart in half
trying not to let you down,
i want to be true to myself
and still keep you around.
why does doing what is right for me
lead to hurting you?
stuck between a rock and a hard place,
i don't know what to do.
when i am being tugged one way
but the opposite leads to you.
regardless of what i choose—
somehow
i still lose.

i wish we knew each other when we were younger.
we could have run through fields together,
aiding days of sorrow with laughter.
we could have shared stories
about our dreaming and confusion.
we could've been there for each other
when the world got loud.
we could have lifted each other up
when the voices of others drowned ours out.
if we had known each other back then,
maybe those children we once were
would've felt a little less lonely.

ebb and flow

i will scribble about you
in coffee shops that exist
in cities you have never been to.

i will get a cramp in my hand
by filling the pages with
every memory of the way we laughed.

it will be repetitive;
the barista will know my name,

and i will recite
as much as i can remember

until you can live on between pages

and i can keep you
where you always were—

stuck in the middle.

our eyes met across the airport terminal,
and through relief-fuelled adrenaline,
i ran as fast as i could to get to you.
when you held me,
i hoped that the embrace
after a decade of waiting
was strong enough
that you would never think about
letting me go
again.

you're the pull that brings me back
every time i drift away.
you're the number i call
when i'm having a bad day.
you're the reason i stay afloat,
the one who knows me most.
what am i going to do
when your time here finally stops?
where am i going to go
when one day you're here
and the next you're not?
without your guidance,
in every decision i'm never sure.
how do i move on with life
when i don't have my magnet anymore?

i reluctantly know that at some point there will be a day that starts without you in it. that day will be followed by an immense amount of firsts: the first time that my heart gets broken and i can't come running to you, the first time that i need your advice but i can't call you, the first hometown visit where i don't sleep over at your house, and the first time i hear jokes that i know would make you laugh that i can't send. it is suffocating, the amount of life that will persist whilst your soul will cease to exist. i can't begin to fathom how the world will continue on when you are gone. i always try to turn a blind eye when the thoughts creep in, but they are hard to shift when the tears begin to stream and the silence becomes piercing. i don't know what i'd do without you. i have never known life to be lived without you. i resent the time that i'll have to. i hope that if there is a being that guides us, they are kind. i hope they are generous with their time before i have to miss you for the rest of my life.

sometimes we need to let go
because the hurt from the loss
is healthier than the hurt
caused by repeating cycles
in dire need of being broken.

i worry that it's too late, that we have passed our prime. i worry that the timing is wrong and we have missed the potential to get this right. i worry that this will be another repeat because i've always known disaster. i worry that the words you say will not match up to your actions after. i worry that i am being gullible to be optimistic for change; i worry that no matter how much i heal it is inevitable that things will end the same. i worry that you will live up to the childhood version of you i curated in my mind. i worry that this is a delusion that will result in how it always ends, where i put my heart in your hands and you leave it behind.

the rain has started pouring,
and i don't know what is next for me.

i used to pride myself on knowing;
i could trust my intuition fearlessly
because if the idea felt right
then i had to see how life would look
from the other side.

but today the rain is heavy,
and my hair is messy,
and i don't know what is next for me.

i know that i don't need to,
nobody *really* knows either.

but i *did* and well,
it got me this far.
so if i do not know now...

where do i go from here?

fall

ebb and flow

*i wonder what it is like to not wonder about
the rest of your life.*

*how the days feel when you aren't thinking about
how everything looks from another side.*

*it must be so calming to not question
if every decision is right.*

*how enjoyable it must be when you aren't
worrying about running out of time.*

i have a habit of thinking about
the worst case scenario.
if things crumble,
where do i run and where can my heart go?
how do i protect myself?
how will i cope with loss
and whatever is left?
i forget that life can work out
if i give it the chance to.
if i run away from everything i have ever wanted
out of fear that it does not want me—

how will i ever get there?

i lied to you when i said i was fine.
i hoped you wouldn't dig deeper
and avoid the warning signs.

i didn't want to be a bother,
or stand in the way
of you focusing on something else
or enjoying your well-deserved sunny days.

i didn't want to admit
that the clouds are getting heavy,
the sky has turned grey
or the waves are no longer steady.

i didn't want you to see
everything bubbling underneath—

because i was scared that
if i opened my mouth,

the floods wouldn't stop

and i'd forget how to breathe.

katie cecilia

i am trying my best
to keep everything together,
appearing to be smooth sailing
to hide my stormy weather.

i know how to perform.
i have done this before,
pretending the weight isn't crushing me
so they don't see my aching bones
and decide they don't want me anymore.

i know this isn't healthy.
i know the habit isn't necessary,
but i always fall back into being
a lifeboat for the drowning
instead of saving myself
when i really need it most.

ebb and flow

you're demanding answers
about exposed bruises
and outdated conversations.
i dance around the subject,
listening with tears streaming in silence.
i can't take another rip
of this worn-down bandage
because if i do not take the time
to process my emotions,
they will show up
where they aren't invited.

it is happening again,
when the world gets loud
and my heart feels heavy.
when my thoughts overflow
but minimal words come out.
it is taking all of me
to function through daily tasks.
i am being gentle with myself
as i wade through this low,
until i can get my spark back.

ebb and flow

i am waiting in this doorway
like all the times before
after years of telling myself
i wouldn't do this anymore.

is it naive or optimistic
to think you'll come home?
when all i have ever done
is carry this weight alone.

i peek around the frame
to check if you're there,
expecting that you would be
when you said that you still care.

i stand here
hoping this time will be the one
where the chance to rebuild with me
means more than how long you were gone.

i talk to my ceiling
hoping it'll get to you
with tears streaming,
a cracking voice pleading
that you'll help me through.
i hope that you hear me,
that i'm not just talking to my ceiling.
i hope life lives on beyond the grave.
i hope you are there
because i don't know what is worse
realising that you're not
or being alone
in this place.

that text message sat in my notes app long after you left. i hoped i could keep it there until you ultimately came back so there would be no leaving to process. it has been years; the note falls lower down the list. apart from the memories in my head, life is starting to look like we didn't exist. if i voiced that i thought of you still, everyone would call me crazy. my heart was never made of steel or clay; *i've never been one to let go easily.*

i never want to clean this room
because
           if i did

                i'd be the only mess left.

nobody tells you how hard leaving your first apartment is. taping boxes filled with memorabilia, impulse purchases and leftover dish soap. how difficult it is to peel away photos and posters, stripping away vibrance and personality to reveal blank, empty walls. how by the time all of your belongings are taken away, it is almost like you were never there at all. there is a moment where you look around, noticing how everything is as bare as it was when you first arrived. the only evidence of living is chipped paint and worn-down stovetops. your absence will leave space for someone new to have somewhere to feel safe in and to create new rituals and rooms to decorate. it is bittersweet to be ready for the horizon of opportunity and growth but to know that getting there costs the first place that gave you independence, the first place that felt like home. nobody talks about how heavy the moment is when you know *you have to let that go.*

tell me
when was it?
the moment you learnt that
a life without me was one you'd prefer.

at what moment did your heart
stop beating for mine?
i can feel your hand slipping
and it is only a matter of time
until i no longer reside in your mind.

i never thought i would
see the day
your eyes stopped holding
that same gaze for me.

even when you are right here
next to me,
we have never been further apart.

i know how being left feels.
just tell me what it was
that made your feelings fade—
so i know that to be loved
i can never be that way.

ebb and flow

every time i visit my hometown,
i hope i'll run into you
in a coffee shop somewhere
or a bus stop with just us two.

i wonder what you'd say
if you saw me all this time later.
would you smile? would you dismiss me?
or say you should've treated me better?

we never really said goodbye—
just faded into the mist
of growing up and collecting distractions,
leaving the back of our minds
as the only place to reminisce.

it is probably delusion
that fuels the hope of seeing you again.
there is just this tiny part of me
that still believes, despite the years;
our story hasn't ended yet.

here i am on this cheap couch
in a room bursting with laughter,
surrounded by faces
that i would die for,
and all my heart can feel
is the lack of you in here.
you chose not to be,
you are wrapped up in sheets
a couple of floors above me,
and it hurts
because this room is filled with love,
and i block it out
because yours
was the only one i wanted.

i'd like to think that somewhere in the parallel we are still friends. we still laugh in the sunlight and notice how the streets twist and bend. in our alternative storylines, neither of us drifts away. we still daydream of being maids of honour and keep each other's secrets safe. there is a place far from here where i call to ask about your day – it is warm and light, and i do not spend every milestone glancing over at your empty space.

it would've been easy to let you back in again. repetition becomes a habit, and habits are comfortable. being used to temperamental crashing waves does not mean that i deserve the chaos. i swim through calmer seas now. the silence is therapeutic. i could have let you visit, but i know now to never trust a storm – especially when they are predicted to be mild when history suggests otherwise.

i couldn't let you go without emptying the contents of the box collecting dust. i clung on to the birthday cards, jar of notes and letters. reading them again only resurfaced the buried sting of you leaving. hoarding keepsakes only ignites the hope that you will come back someday. the scraps of the past give me reassurance that we existed, but holding onto them keeps my growth on a leash. i poured them all out and read each one until i mustered the courage to throw them away. this is how i'm saying goodbye, on the bedroom floor of a new apartment two years later in a city that you don't live in anymore.

suppressing does not dissolve the feelings,
the pressure will only lead you to erupt.

ebb and flow

little me cried when she talked about you,
older me does too.
even when we do the work to heal,
sometimes,
we still drown in shades of blue.

there have been nights where i have rewritten our
last conversation out of hindsight. you never
returned, and if i had known that then i would
not have held back. i was convinced this was our
usual rodeo; i treated you leaving as such. how
foolish that my dependence on our cycles would
lead to us never speaking again.

it always comes when you least expect it, when you're trying to heal from it or run away from it altogether. grief does not schedule an appointment, and triggers do not care for suitable times and preferred displays of emotion. there is not a designated room to release built-up energy or any slot allocated for processing reminders and grovelling your reality. life continues to move forward, and tomorrow will be another day regardless of what time your world stopped or where you misplaced your soul. my head is drifting, and my heart is screaming, and i remind myself that *feelings were created to be felt*. when they are, they arrive abruptly and inconveniently; they fade away, leaving trails of exhaustion and guilt from another day of juggling the emotional phases and holding myself together in hopes of not spilling over the rim of my mental bucket. it feels inappropriate to take shelter, even when i can hear my eardrums warning me to catch my breath. i cannot be oblivious to the piercing silence, no matter how much i deny its appearance or wish i could be. whilst i usually promote floating through gentle shallow waters and soft-spoken rainfall, *i am drowning in mine.*

i don't know how to tell you
that i need an apology to move on,
how i can't brush past your temperament
and how it made me become.
i'm scared of being honest
even though that is all i want.
for years i have cradled
this aching heart
and i still haven't figured out
how to make it stop.

ebb and flow

my chances wear thin eventually
like my childhood favourite shoes.
with usage, they get weaker until
there isn't enough left to be functional.
for you,
i would superglue and redesign entirely
but i can't ignore the ripped stitches
or the puddles that soak through.

i am a glass made for pouring—
always placed waiting to serve.
every drop preowned.
when you began to pour into me,
i had no choice
but to fall apart on the kitchen counter.
no one has ever returned what i gave.
no one cared about the empty glass
who always gave
what she never had.

how ironic is it that we feel lonely in the experiences where we are not alone? this is universal, the push and pull of growing up. when the voice in your head gets loud, it is common to forget that it isn't the only one speaking. even when you are quiet. even when you do not want to talk about it. you are not alone. your hurt and happiness are felt in more than your heart. you belong. you are never by yourself in the experience of renewal and rust.

if you need proof of this,

i am right there with you.

i am still working to undo
the patterns you put me through.

unravelling beliefs
that remain untrue
about who you said i'd become
and all the damage you swore i'd do.

i am not the person
you painted me out to be.

you knew i was good,
i knew i was good

and you knew

you had to take that from me.

every now and then, i forget
that i haven't been a child
for some time.
there is nobody coming to get me
to place me back on my feet.
where i go
relies solely on my own movement.
i get to read the map
to plan my own journey.

how exciting—
that the world has opened up.
how lonely—
that the hand to hold is gone
now i am deemed old enough
to no longer need it.

nostalgia is a liar. she sweetens every sour moment
just enough to make me question if it was ever *that*
bad; she highlights and underlines the good times so
that when i am reminiscing, i begin to miss those
moments. there are reasons that i do not live there
or have those people around me anymore. i have to
remind myself of the ugly, the thunderstorms and
the cracks in my heart that are still mending. i have
to remind myself of all the good i have now and to
put the phone down. i have to be vigilant because
she is such a good storyteller, and i am a sucker for
a happy ending.

someday
remembering you will wash over me
and i'll rinse the memories away.
like soap on skin
you will not stick.
instead,
i will appreciate
everything that you did
and be thankful
that you will never be able
to stain again.

surge

ebb and flow

it does not matter
how far you run
if you do not befriend and heal your ghosts
they will follow you
wherever you go.

the water rises around my lungs,
almost enough to suffocate the air out of them,
inch by inch, the more i try to swim.
splashes catch my eyes—
deep breaths,
vision blurred,
and yet i keep treading.
the calm has come before,
the tides will slow,
there will be stillness.
i will be able to float again

i am always in a rush.

to scale the next mountain for a prettier, more satisfying view, until i notice a glimpse of the neighbouring mountain with a steeper rock surface bathed in brighter sunrises, and once again, i am on the move. today is all we are promised; i place an egg in every basket out of panic that if i do not try to simultaneously live the contrasting experiences i crave, time will not be so kind, and i will blink and be double my age with a pocket of regrets and even less than i started with. i have defined my worth with my achievements and what i am capable of so deeply that being categorised in a tick box makes me claustrophobic, and stillness makes me homesick. i have a mind that races and a heart with pieces scattered in many places. the more dreams that manifest, the more longing i do, the space expands, and i scramble to occupy it with busy schedules and appeasing antidotes that i hope nobody sees through. oftentimes the wildflowers and farmland tend to go unseen as my eyes fixate on the next sunset on the horizon, always out of reach.

my fear of being perceived
has limited my ability to evolve
for a century.
i desperately want my world view to expand
but the notion is mortifying
that to attain acknowledgement
i have to uncover softness
that has spent years
buried underneath.

ebb and flow

i am sat at a desk,
with a spinning office chair,
daydreaming about cities
i haven't been to yet
and reminiscing about
the ones i have.

i do not wish to sit
with a brick wall window view
until my spine arches,
and i have nothing to show for
the life i was blessed with.

my writings are scattered
across a book, and my notes app,
and i don't know
if it will ever become more than that.

but as long as i sit here,
with my wrists placed on hickory panelling,

i will think about how
i want to be creating and exploring
instead of scheduling meetings
that could've been emails,
and pouring into a world
that will only take from me.

i wonder if i will ever see the world
get on a plane and just
leave.
i'm good at leaving.
i've left many people
because if i leave then i cannot be left.
if i was to be left
i would know that i was worth leaving
and if i know that
i wouldn't ever want someone to stay.
so i leave,
when they love me,
when they want me.
because if i leave
then i cannot be left
and if i leave,
i don't need to watch them fall out of love with me
because if i can fall out of love with me
they can too
so i tell them it's me,
not them
and i leave
because if i leave, then i cannot be left.

i hope i can get to a point where i am not shouting at voids and ringing bells at closed hearts to be heard. i hope i can reach a place where i don't feel the need to justify every decision and dissect my entire life when they chastise me for trying. i hope i can get there, to a place where i live my life as unapologetically and categorically me as possible.

i thought i would always have one more moment
with you,
that there was an abundance of time
to be in your company.
i took every moment for granted,
from assuming i would get another.
it is only now, when your existence is only visible
in the memories i rehearse
that i realise
just how magical those days we spent together were.
i should've noticed it sooner,
but there is nothing i can do
but hold tight to every reminder
and let the sky know
just how much i miss you.

we are like water
how we return to each other in waves.
we crash over and over
as the climate begins to change.
flowing down canals,
wiping away our beloved streets
even when we drown neighbourhoods
we still cannot give each other what we need.

this time i am leaving with a heavier heart than before. i finally see how high i've climbed, and now i am wishing i was still on the floor. i am reminded of how many ages i wished away to get here in hopes that as i got older, the way i saw the world would become clear. i feel conned; all i did increase the number. i have never been more connected to myself, but my loved ones and i couldn't be more distant from each other. i don't have my next steps lined up; what lies before me is a blur. i want to run back to my teenage self and shake her shoulders. being rich was about what she held, and despite the pressures and dictators, there was never anything wrong with her.

my future self will find me washed up on the shore of our hometown and tell me why i made the right choice. she will thank me for following my intuition and show me the highs she has seen. she will come to get me. she is the only one who understands the depths we have been to. she will hold my hand and tell me everything will be okay. i know she will because i visit my past all of the time.

i am heading back to my hometown. everything feels familiar, but everything has changed. the streets have post boxes and cobbled paths like they used to, but i am not nineteen, nor will i ever be again. there is no comfort like being at my mother's place, but nothing feels the same. there is nowhere i'd rather be, but my heart does not live there anymore. when i leave, i miss the familiarity. when i stay, the memories are suffocating. there will never be a place that knows me the way those walls do. they will never know the extent of who i become. being away has made me free of everything but the nostalgia of feeling whole somewhere. i cannot shake the bitter reality. i am outgrowing where i grew, each visit teaches me that this place will never be able to hold me the way it used to.

what if i do not live up to
the super star title from my mother?
what if the path i choose doesn't work,
and i wish i had picked another?
what if my dreams never make it
during my loved ones lifetime?
what if despite my intentions,
i'm not able to get this right?
what if everything i try to make turns to dust?
what if everyone in the rooms i walk into
realises that i am not good enough?
what if the ball drops
because something always seems to give.
what if i *can't*
or i *stop*
and whatever talent i do have,
i am too late to do anything with?
what if i lose out?
what if i am in my own way?
what if i spend years running
only to find that nothing stays the same?
why do i have to be so passionate
but be fearful of change?
why is the thought of not being great
reason enough
for my self-belief to dissipate?

i am starting to doubt the decisions i swore by.
if i am not that person, then who am i?
if i do not know myself,
how am i supposed to explain it to anyone else?
i have never been this confused.
i was so sure.
how can i just wake up on a sunny day and realise
i no longer wish for the heat anymore?

there has been a shift in the air
i don't feel terrible
but i don't feel great, either.
catastrophe and inconvenience
usually warrant feelings like these.
not much has changed
but i have
and yet, i do not know
what caused this
or where to put
my empty heart.

i have sat with indecision,
dissecting every move i could make
conflicted as to which would be
the "right" one.

i have done this many times
out of fear of regretting my actions,
judgement from others,
and the opinion of my future self.

and yet, even now—
after all my investigative attempts
and nervous choices—
the worrisome regret
for the things i did
has never seeped in.

the only regret i could have
is that i didn't make decisions
when my gut was screaming.

the only regret i could have
is how long it took
to trust myself.

ebb and flow

you think you'll never write again
until you pick up the pen.
you think you'll never feel better
until now turns into back then.
you think that things will never change
until you notice the shift.
you think you're stuck under the weight
until the pressure begins to lift.
you think you'll never find love
until you learn your first has to be you.
you think that nothing will improve
until you put in the work
and realise, they always do.

reflect

ebb and flow

my mother is moving house
she is keeping my childhood bed
maybe this means i can hang on
to my youth
for a little longer.

laying between childhood bedsheets,
i begin to revisit
every age i have ever been
and the places i still miss.
i am much taller now—
my feet reach the end of the bed.
i haven't been seventeen for a while
but somehow,
those feelings haven't left yet.
it is strange to grow up
but not grow out of the years before.
my pillow collects every thought
letting me know i am always welcome
even when i am not young anymore.

my therapist does not tell me
which direction to go.
she listens
and asks questions
as i find the answers myself.
as i navigate my mind,
i learn
that the answers live within us.
sometimes,
we just need someone
with a flashlight
to help us search for them.

the traumas and woes of your relatives are theirs
to carry and dissect. you can hold hands. you can
pour out affirmations with love harmonies, but it
is not up to you to put the pieces back together or
do the work for anyone who is not willing to take
the necessary steps to heal their hurt.

ebb and flow

if everyone around you
is choosing to take part
in the hurtful hereditary cycles
then maybe
the needed change
is meant to start with you.

you are not a bad person
for not emptying every thought
at the dining room table.
you can choose what you share
and who you share it with.
you may feel all out of options
but one will always remain.
you are allowed to pick
what streams parts of yourself
flow into.

when i was twelve,
i went to therapy for the first time.
i sat across from a woman;
she was brunette with a soft smile,
and she didn't try to fix my life.
she did not dictate.
she sat there and heard me,
asked sporadic questions
and gave me the space
to pour out to her.
i cried many times in that chair;
she only ever saw me tear-stained.
from those days with her,
i learnt that
i did not need someone
to pick up my pieces.
i just needed a place
where my hurting heart
would feel
listened to.

here i am again,
mourning a future
i never even wanted
because disappearing in any success
would have been better than nothing.

this feels like endlessly spinning
through revolving doors,
from getting everything i wanted
to it not being what i want anymore.

i need to remind myself
that it isn't a loss
if i didn't want it.

a closed door
does not mean that others
are not already open,
waiting for me.

healing is reversing into the driveway of the house you moved out of a very long time ago just to have one more moment of familiarity. you shouldn't be there, but you sit. you've already left this driveway before. you know you can again, and you will – but it's a tuesday night and you heard the song that you both used to sing along to and you just needed one more cry on the kerb. you take a look around as you put the keys in the ignition and swear that it's the last time you'll leave this driveway. you know better. it has been so long. you eventually begin to turn the wheels, smearing your tears and avoiding looking in the rear-view mirror. you will do this over and over, months and years apart. you don't know when the next time will be, but with each visit, you'll be there less and less. until it becomes just another driveway that you think of but no longer make the journey to.

katie cecilia

after years of running,
i sat by the lake and admitted defeat.

the waters continued to flow,
the sun stayed lighting the sky,
the earth would continue on
whether i strived forward
or buried my head in the dirt.

the world would not wait for me
to get back on my feet.
i could have stayed sitting there,
waiting for a sign to move forward,
or i could begin by walking slowly each day
toward where i needed to be.

if nothing would pause
then i needed to get going—
even if my pace was gradual,
nature would accompany me.

the rain and i are friends tonight; she is streaming down in the lamplight, and mine are dancing down my skin, reflecting in my eyes. i am doing everything i can to keep it all together, but there is a constant cloud of paranoia following me, telling me all of the ways i could do it all better. i am trying. i am trying my best. if the rain can subside for sunlight, i can't give up just yet.

being anxious about something
is not a weakness.
wanting something to go well
and wanting things to work out
is a positive attribute to have.
rather than throwing
caution to the wind,
you take something important to you
like a box of fragile glasses
and you handle it
with care.

nobody is mad at you. nobody is going to tell you off. you are an adult now. you can do what you want. they can say what they like. they no longer get to decide. you are leading in your own life, and unlike what you may have been told, you are allowed to change your mind. they may have gotten to control you once. they do not get to anymore. you have made it to the other side, honey; this life is finally *yours.*

now that i'm older
i understand why seasons change—
how learning in hindsight grows
the more that you age.
i understand
how prolonged winters
can leave you bitter,
how the sunsetting
does not mean it will forever.
now that i have grown
i understand the change in weather—
but the little girl
who lives within
she deserved better.

i am starting to feel my younger self slipping away. i still have a version of her, but she doesn't feel the same way. i used to be on the phone talking for hours into the night, and now my bedtime is much earlier, and i no longer sleep with a light. the chaotic last-minute plans and gossiping sessions are now scheduled coffee dates months in advance and comparing life lessons. i can feel my days turning from exhilarating curiosity to comfortable flows. i mostly enjoy this change, but i am not ready to let her go. they say to enjoy the moments while they last; you don't realise how fast they are going to go. i dismissed their words back then, but now i wish i could go back in time and let her know. i am in my twenties; there is still so much room for exploration left. there will be joy and tears and well-needed rest. my life isn't over; it's just starting to look different than before. i wish i had known that they were the "good old days" before her youth wasn't mine anymore.

the fickle and fearful version of myself
is the person that got me here.
she weathered chaotic storms
and wiped tears from sore eyes.
i owe her everything
for the sunrises i see now
which is why
it is gut-wrenching
to sit in this therapy chair
and know
it is time to let her go.

ebb and flow

please do not live your life
bypassing opportunities
out of expecting them to always be there.
time changes everything.
our perceptions shift.
what you have today
could be entirely different tomorrow.
when you have the chance
to see that person, go to that place
or have that experience.
please go for it.
do not leave your future self
to live with wishing
they had taken the leap
that you can
right now.

it is never too late to be better. it will not change the past. bitterness can be hard to shake, but you can evolve; you can actively choose to improve every day. it is going to be hard. it is going to be challenging. to get to the greener grass, you have to start watering your own. your dedication to nurturing is the only way that someday flowers will grow.

ebb and flow

i will not forgive everything you did,
but i will place the weight on the grass i watered.
i will not carry you through
everywhere i go next.
you do not deserve compassion
but i deserve more
than a man that persists
to remind my sunny skies
of every rainy day.

katie cecilia

i know the love i yearn for exists
because it burns inside me
and in the hands of so many
who did not deserve
to bask in its warmth.

outgrowing the place that raised me is bittersweet,
those same streets still hold people
i care about deeply.
the green bench that hosted
all of my starry teenage nights
still sits in the park
that my mothers place is nearby.
a town with low ceilings is no match for me—
my mind always wanders to where else i could be.
the drifting has led me far,
my dreams never seem to lack—
but through my chasing
i did not mean for the city i adored
to be the same one
i would stop wanting back.

staying is a valid option too. planting your life next to your favourite streets with those you love can be healing. tangling your roots somewhere that you feel cared for can make you rich. staying creates memories and layers of knowing each other. those layers can unravel years of stories that are long overdue to be rewritten. staying can create a home. staying can create comfort zones. staying can create love. the media and ideals of others can say otherwise. if being rooted feels right to you, staying is good enough too.

ebb and flow

you will never know this version of me
and that is a shame
because i have healed in ways
beyond what i knew.
i am at peace with myself,
my heart has space.
if only you hadn't been so reckless,
a chair at my table
could've been carved with your name.

i know there is no timeline
and that i have years on my side
to decide what i want to do with this life.
i simply fear that
if my dreams are not reached
in a youthful body with eyes to see
and lungs to breathe,
the time i spent chasing
things that i never wanted
will catch up with me.
i fear if i wait long enough,
the wrinkles and priorities will stack,
and i will be left wondering what could've been
if i did not tell myself to slow down
or hold myself back.

it is so scary to look in the mirror and see my adult self when there is a child inside me that is still processing and healing. i want to wrap her up in cotton wool and never let anything bad happen to her (*again*) but i can't. i move forward and drag my feet every birthday in hopes that it'll slow the process down and i can hang on tight to the strands of my youth for a little while longer.

(i miss her already, and she hasn't even left yet.)

i know that even if i could halt time to absorb these moments for a few minutes more, i would be holding her back. if she knew about where life has led us this far, she would be screaming, dancing and begging for the footnote details. she would be smiling ear to ear as i recite how we saw our favourite band for the first time or how we found love again. she would be in awe of all we achieved despite the heavily opinionated tones around her telling her otherwise. she would want to be me. she would want me to continue to see what life has to offer and someday come back to tell her all about it. she would want us to live it, to see where all of the ups and downs lead to.

younger me, i'm doing this for you.

we spend so much time honing in on our goals and ticking a checkbox that we often forget that *these are the moments we once begged for.* these are the moments that we burnt out and sacrificed sleep for. oftentimes i have to remind myself of where i am standing and the amount of climbing and reflection it has taken to even recognise myself in the mirror again. i put excessive amounts of pressure on myself to outrun my potential; that *far* is never far enough. i have to remind myself to stop tugging on my training wheels, that it is okay if my journey needs a brisk commute around the houses for a while. i remind myself that breaks are important; a slingshot will only travel a great distance if it is pulled back enough. i used to wish to be able to breathe, to be someone who could decide for herself and to have people around me who authentically raise me up. to be blessed with options and to have the strength to become better. it is easy for me to get fixated on the goalposts that the surrounding area seems blurry. even when i am nowhere near the next target, even in the moments where i am not running or climbing, the person who i am today is not only who will take me wherever i am supposed to go next—*she is the person i yearned to be.*

being in my twenties has taught me how intense it feels to experience every emotion all at once, to look back and laugh at silly childhood photographs and memories. to scribble all of my dreams down excitedly in this year's diary, which are the complete opposite from what they were the year before. to make decisions only to doubt them and contradict them. to lie awake at night thinking of every person that once meant something to me, being relieved i made it through and trying to ignore the slight tear in my heart any time i remember tender moments or unticked bucket lists. the twenties have been undeniably loud, with plenty to store away, unpack and be excited for. the twenties have made it clear to me that emotions are multifaceted and that the human experience is complex. the chaos of storms is usually found in the aftermath, especially when you have been in hiding in bunkers for too long. the twenties have embodied what it is to feel, to reflect and to let go—after all of the years when all i wanted to do was fade away, it is liberating to know that i got to feel the beauty of self-connection because i chose to stay.

strength is not only the ability to carry heavy weight;
it is also knowing
when it is time to leave,
time to seek help,
and time to put yourself first.

strength is more than suffering and success.
strength is the in-between decisions too.

ebb and flow

the crippling pressure you put on yourself to outdo every goal you set is rotting your soul. slow down and watch the ocean. sip your favourite drink and hold hands with someone you love. our limited time here is meant to be predominantly enjoyed. these days are not a punishment. you will not hold every achievement, but not every room will have the honour of holding you. pursue what your heart beats for and know this, *being everything for everyone all of the time will never be a requirement for you to deserve a place in this world.*

some days are made for crying to sad movies and moving a little slower. the world still rotates; today is yet again another saturday but for some reason all my heart wants to do is hide under a heap of blankets and pretend for one moment that existence has paused and that i can catch up. days like this are exhausting despite how little movement actually happens. joy and celebration shout muffled positive affirmations and well wishes, but somehow i still walk in circles under my thought raincloud. with every hour that passes by, i sit rotting on this couch; my mind has never felt this dry, yet if it were to rain today, i fear that i may drown entirely. days like this are long, difficult and heavy. i am glad i can feel intensely; eventually i will feel the contrast. this much depth can hold light too; these days are not what i wish for but what i need. i'll take time to build an umbrella; all of this weather can only lead to rainbows.

ebb and flow

the space i created
between you and i
did not diminish the love
i had for you.
it was to protect my heart
from being mishandled
and broken again
at the hands
of you.

katie cecilia

as much as i wish
we could have happened sooner,
i am grateful for how everything unfolded,
because the timing allowed us
to be mature enough
and emotionally ready
to handle the weight
of how glorious
a life with each other can be
when we learn
to grow together.

ebb and flow

maybe those dreams weren't mine.
maybe my voice was under hypnosis,
acting as an echo
of what i was taught.

the views and pursuits
that were labelled as noble
in the eyes of those
that looked like mine.

but the clouds and fog have cleared.
my outlook has shifted.

maybe the *world* is much bigger.
maybe there *is* much more.
maybe *i* could be much more—

more than they ever said i could be,
more than i ever thought i could be.

you are not obligated to stay anywhere
that is not serving you anymore.

you can let go of dreams
if they are no longer
what you reach for.

your definition of success can be reinvented.
everything changes
all of the time.
take this as a sign
that you can too.

ebb and flow

i have seen what staying there does—
to be deeply wrapped up in the past
that you miss what is right in front of you.
how the years fly by
from waiting in hope for an alternative ending
through gripping on to moments we cannot change.

i fear losing out on any more days this way.

i want to actively be here—
present,
open and forthcoming.

i do not know what will come next, but i know this:

i will do the work to be *here*
by making peace with what happened *there*.

even though this next chapter
erupts with joy,
i will still be sad
about the loss it took
to receive such solitude.

release

new starts can make you sad. you can be excited about what is to come and still mourn what you had. every time i turn a new leaf, i still miss old ones that have become rotten or drifted away. i have reminisced while also being relieved that aspects of my life changed. like a coin, you can have both sides. that doesn't mean you shouldn't do it; that doesn't mean you shouldn't try. even some of our happiest times greet us with an element of goodbye.

take a deep breath.
lower your shoulders.
unclench your jaw.
stop
just for a minute.
allow yourself some time
to take a mental break.
you cannot carry all things.
you are doing enough.
you are enough.
you can give, if you must
but keep a minute,
or two,
for you.

soul searching can result in
only your footprints for a while.
step forward anyway.
the company you wait for
may never come.
proceed. reach. arrive.
anyone who will intertwine
will be waiting to greet you
on the other side.

ebb and flow

take off your coat,
hang it on the door.
you don't need a plan
or have everything figured out at all.
you can take up a hobby,
you can get more sleep,
you can try each day
focusing on what you need.
it may not be tomorrow,
or someday soon,
but one day,
you will learn
that the way you live is enough
even when sometimes,
it only makes sense to you.

my loneliness taps me on the shoulder
to remind me of all our empty space.
i sigh with relief and say:

"look how much room we have
for the sunny days to arrive.
we will not need to excuse the mess.
we will be able to celebrate
every magical moment
and feel comfortable
in the rearranging".

i see the potential
in how we look at each other,
in how we laugh,
in how the memories make you light up
and how we overlap.
i see the hypotheticals dance in my head
from all of the possibilities
we have left.
i am hoping it is not a fantasy.
i hope this time
the potential becomes our reality
because this time
it is us
starting again.

when you find healthy love
for the first time,
you feel sick—

because you're grateful
that they're here.

but now you know:

it was *that easy.*

it was that easy,
and they still treated you that way.

when you find healthy love
for the first time,
it's two things:

immersing yourself
in their love—

and healing
from who didn't.

i am still learning to trust kindness,
to bask in the sun
without expecting to burn.
it is taking me a while,
i have come a long way
but i need more time
for my reluctancy
to turn into peace.

i knew you loved me
when i could feel it in the way you listened,
in the way you remembered
the *just because* gestures.

you accepted every corner of my life,
even the parts that collect dust.

i knew you loved me
when you showed me how far you would go,
you sat next to me patiently as i unraveled
and rebuilt who i wanted to be.

i knew you loved me
when i realised that i had never really been *loved* before
there was no facade or expectation.

you intertwined your life in between my lines,
this was lightweight,
this was *"we will figure it out together"*
this was home being a person.

i knew you loved me
because i never had to wonder if you did.

the person i was before you did not believe that i deserved a love like this; she was convinced that adoration came with a price to pay, and she stacked boxes and walls to stop hopeful butterflies from creeping in. she would never let the thoughts build; there was risk in creation, and she feared hyper-fixating on a life that only fairytales show and would avoid the slightest temptation. the person i was before you had her guard up; she would deflect and contrast your palette to appear as though it wouldn't work. she would pick at your potential and deny all feelings to avoid being hurt. the person i was before was terrified of meeting you someday; the devil you know is always more comfortable, and since calmness was foreign territory, she assumed you would break her in the same way. when that person finally met you, she would hide how she daydreamed of us being together; she would refuse your sunshine since she was accustomed to foggy weather. the person i was before you needed you to break through the myths and theories of what love could truly be. she needed you to bypass the traps and tricks so she could realise that there was reason in the madness—that it all happened *so you could find me.*

you are going to outgrow versions of yourself and people that you thought you would keep forever. change moulds us day by day; oftentimes the person you were a year ago is drastically different from who you are now and you realise in hindsight but don't always notice the gradual altering. there are moments where the shoes just don't fit you anymore, places don't feel how they used to and someone you know becomes someone you knew. these things are inevitable; they are not always a result of rash decisions or arguments. there are times when their direction shifts, your view of your horizon expands and you both embark on new adventures. give yourself the time to grieve what you have lost, but know that absence creates space for new beginnings.

even after years of repair and therapy, i still have days of despair. i still wake up sick from remembering and second-guessing everything around me. there is not a timeline for working on yourself. there isn't an ultimate test or specific day where the back and forth in my mind will be put to rest. each day is a choice to be better. each day is an opportunity to learn a different perspective. the ache softens, but hard days still exist. they appear as days and not weeks like they once were. the progress is still evident, even when the difficult feelings resurface.

katie cecilia

for the first time
i'm not thinking about how much i weigh
or the food on my plate.
i'm laughing and dancing
with a smile on my face.
i'm not worrying about how i am perceived
or anybody else.
this is the beginning
of finding my way
back to myself.

it is only now,
when i am reaching my
mid-twenties,
that i feel i'm meeting myself.

that is not to say
i did not know myself previously.
there were versions i loved,
versions i liked,
and versions, well...
out of sight, out of mind.

now that i have the freedom to decide
alongside the stubbornness
to be adamant in what i like,
it feels like i am holding hands
with my soul.

no facade to impress,
no masks or fancy dress.
just me, enjoying what makes me tick.

it is nice to finally find peace
in not having all of the pieces fit.

you are a mosaic of everything you have experienced. you have a glow from the sunset you saw on that one trip. you have sweetness from your first taste of ice cream. your laughter from that one day with your friends brightens the dullest of skies. your softness from your empathy towards a lover creates the most comforting shades. you are not just what you have hurt from; you are every good thing you have lived through, too.

i spent a really long time convinced that my life belonged somewhere else. that wherever i was standing was nothing in comparison to how i could hypothetically be living. on occasion, those moments motivated me to change aspects of my life but by the time i had made the changes, i was thinking about a new version of my reality entirely. i lost many days this way. we are not promised anything. all we have is the time we are given, and as ambitious as my mind is, there is no accomplishment like taking the opportunity to be present where i am. i am learning to not get lost in the clouds, that i will never get anywhere if i am everywhere, and that time will pass no matter where i am. i am learning to absorb what surrounds me. i will never get this back.

your twenties are not the best years of your life.
they are not the years of knowing it all
or getting everything right.
these are the years of trial,
a constant remeasure of your pieces and how they fit.
these are the beginner days of creating your own life
and learning how to manage it.
there are an abundance of options
and even more decisions to make.
there is no universal timing,
take this journey at your own pace.
enjoy the good moments but rest assured,
there is more to come.
these years have turbulence and confusion
so when you feel it, you aren't the only one.
do not constrict yourself to a timeline,
the future holds extensive space
and trust that through your exploration,
everything will gradually fall into place.

ebb and flow

i don't remember feeling
some of the things i have written about.
that is the beauty of living,
it overlaps and overcomes.
even if it the weight feels heavy for a while
eventually
it gets lighter.

moving on does not mean
that you will never think of them again.
moving on means
moving *forward,*
looking ahead,
and not at what lingers back there.
because your future
is in front of you
and what was
should be kept
exactly where it was left
behind you.

we had to let each other go
to avoid holding each other back
but just know,
i think of you often.
i hope you reach your dreams.
you were always brave.
you can do this
and i can too,
just on different paths
in different ways.

katie cecilia

when the doors burst open
and invite you in,
please walk through.
let go of what has been.
even when it is scary,
even if it's a risk,
grant yourself permission
to explore something different.
if the view isn't what you hoped for
you can always turn around.
but if you never enter the rooms
you'll never find out.

eventually, in your healing journey,
you will reach a crossroads—
where you can let the bitterness consume you,
or you can step forward openly.
either has challenges,
either has benefits.
but when the time comes,
i hope you decide that
where you are going
and the person you are becoming
are so much more important
than whatever came before.

before you lose sight of yourself again
look how far you have come.
notice the perseverance it took
for you to be where you are today.
there is a past version of you somewhere
in awe of everything you have become.
there are always other directions to go
but right now, you are here.
acknowledge that,
sit in this moment.
because no matter what is next
your present self
is worth celebrating too.

i do not silence her anymore,
i let her take up space.
wherever i go
she will know she is safe.
i will not minimise her feelings
to avoid facing her truth
that for us to heal
she needs to be heard too.

-my inner child

there will always be a reason to wait
for days with more sun,
for less weight on our bones,
for months with more money,
and for when wounds have healed from time alone.
but tomorrow may not have space for me,
and you may not see it either.
i will not wait until it is too late
to overflow softness into you,
showing up and shouting
about the ways you captivate me
and give purpose to the things i do.
i will not let time dictate
how much of me you get,
or regret the words i did not say
when we have no moments left.
i give you all of me
even when it is scary to do so.
those moments we wait for may never come;
my love is clear and vibrant,
so you will always know.

i will inevitably scrape my knee multiple times
in this lifetime,
but the ability to stand back up,
despite broken skin and scars,
is what makes the healing process quicker each time.
the wounds may not have been deserved,
the timing may be jagged,
but my light will not be dimmed.
my kindness will only grow,
with each misstep.
i will be stronger and softer,
over and over.

i used to view healing as a milestone to achieve, that when i finally tied pretty bows on everything i loved and cleaned up the mess, that i would feel whole and regenerated. i assumed that the heaviness would grow lighter forever, that these wounds would not serve as reminders because, like my potential, they would fade with time. that is not how anything works. the memories wrapped around my heart become loose until they are tightened once more by the passing smell of perfume or a joke i shared with a friend once. i float until i fall and dust my knees to get up again. there is smoother sailing, but the waves are never calm for long. i feel better than i used to, but there are always tides that rise to make me remember. the hurt lessens, and softness is not permanent; there is a balance to navigating the ocean, and eventually peace can be persistent, if you let it.

ebb and flow

i know how hard you're trying,
and how heavy your days must be,
but i want you to know
how proud i am of you
and how much you mean to me.
i will tell you every day,
until the day you hear it—
i will tell you that
you are enough,
you are worth it,
you are beautiful,
and you deserve to be here,
until you believe it.
take each day,
one moment at a time.
check in with yourself—
you are safe,
you do not need to lie.
there is nowhere else you should be,
this is your journey,
and i am here if you need me.

there are people out there
begging to the sky to meet someone
just like you.
there is a seat at a table
patiently waiting in a room
that you are going to walk into.
there is space for you,
there are places for you
and you don't even know
how close you are
to reaching them.

you will never understand the extent
that your existence morphed my heart
into believing again.
you will never truly know
the healing you enacted
on my scattered mind.
i will tell you anyway
over and over,
as our hair begins to grey
how remarkable your soul is.
because through the adventure
of being loved by you,
i am lucky enough to know
how a heart feels
when it is whole.

rewriting the narrative means
learning to stop rereading previous chapters.

carry the lessons into what you write next,
leave the hurt where it happened.

do not stay there so long
that you confuse
rehearsal for your reality.

maybe my words do not live inside me. maybe they rest there, waiting for their time to leave and find the people they were meant for. i speak to share. i write to release. those acts feel personal when i do them but maybe it was never about me. this whole time, maybe my words served a larger purpose. to be set free to find the soul that needs to hear them.

sit in your emotions long enough to feel them,
but not deep enough that you get stuck there.
blinkers block out light.
you deserve to see how far you've come,
even if the sunlight stings sometimes.

if time won't slow down, and i will never be able to catch up with it. i will hold hands with my loved ones and bask in it. i will bake blueberry muffins and be kind where i go. i will do my best to show up and help people feel less alone. if i will never be able to stop the world spinning so i have a minute to catch my breath. i will get up to dress my bed and face the day with my best when that is both a hundred or twenty-five percent.

the current is unpredictable. the calm may be met with crashes moments later. the ripples may become tsunamis or may stay as low tides approaching the shoreline. there are indicators of change, but these are not definite. the earth only knows impact from what happens—not what *may* happen. this is how i know that the worries in my head are not certain. the collection of water in my bucket will only be held as long as the holes are patched up. i can only control what i know to be true. i can only hold what i have the ability to carry. how i balance the flow is my choice. i can prepare with waterproofs and faith—after that, *i'll look out for the waves.*

let's normalise reaching out
to a friend or a therapy chair.
it is not a weakness to lose sight of the light
and not know how to get there.
it is okay to ask for help,
it is understandable if you do.
you were never supposed to carry it all.
it takes a handhold sometimes
to help you back up
if you fall.

katie cecilia

the eggshells crack on steel pans;
they do not end up on hardwood floors here.
i do not need to tiptoe.
i run down the hallway laughing with my lover.
there is dancing and writing
with long mornings under covers.
i am holding out my hands
towards my younger self to tell her
her storms will subside,
and when they begin to,
everything starts getting better.

if you find yourself making excuses
because someone has potential
please leave.
there is a reason they are not the person
who you think they could be
because if they wanted to,
they would be that person
without you on your knees
begging them to be.

if you stick around
the sun will peek through the clouds
and you will feel the heat on your skin.
if you stay
for a moment more
tomorrow could hold
everything you have asked for.
if you give yourself
one more day
you will get to see
how *everything* can change.

i keep going
for the little girl inside of me
who had no idea
that getting this far
would ever be a possibility for us.

i will not let what has happened to me make me silent or small or timid or hide behind a wall. i will not become mean spirited from all of the weight that i have inherited.

i will be better.

i will be *kind.*

♡ thank you note ♡

this book would not exist without these wonderful people:

my book cover artist, Rosie Rowell (@rosierowell_art):
Thank you for bringing my vision to life with your
gorgeous ocean art. It was lovely to work with you on
the cover of this collection. You are incredibly talented!

my book editors, Tell Tell Poetry (www.telltellpoetry.com):
Thank you for taking the time to edit this collection, your
guidance and advice transformed the way I told the stories
within these poems. I'm so grateful for your careful
attention to detail and your belief in this project.

my loved ones: Thank you to my friends, partner and
family for your unwavering support for my art. You have
brought magic into my life that I never knew was
possible.

&

Thank *you* for being here.

you can find more of my work at @katiececiliapoetry on tiktok and instagram.

www.katiececiliapoetry.com

Published in 2025 in the UK by
Katie Cecilia.

Kindle Direct Publishing.

ISBN: 978-1-83654-521-7

Printed in Dunstable, United Kingdom

70276393R00088